NON GOVERNMENTAL ORGANISATIONS IN HEALTHCARE SERVICE

Practices and Challenges

Karanam Viswa Bhushan

GYAN

Published, 2020

Published by

Gyan Publishing House
5, Ansari Road
Daryaganj, New Delhi-110002
Phone: 011-47034999, 9811692060
www.gyanbooks.com
E-mail: books@gyanbooks.com

Printed at: Gyan Press, Delhi.

Cataloging in Publication Data—DK
Courtesy: D.K. Agencies (P) Ltd. <docinfo@dkagencies.com>

Bhushan, Karanam Viswa, 1963- **author.**
Non governmental organisations in healthcare service : practices and challenges / Karanam Viswa Bhushan.
pages cm
Includes bibliographical references.
ISBN 9788121220286 (HB)

1. Medical care—Ethiopia—Tigray Region. 2. Non-governmental organizations—Ethiopia—Tigray Region. I. Title.

LCC RA410.55.E8B48 2021 | DDC 362.10963 23

Ackowledgments

I would like to thank and express my special glory to the Almighty God.

I sincerely thank for the continuous efforts and involvement of the student Kiflom Gebreselassie Atsebeha.

I would like to extend my gratitude to the personnel of various Non-governmental organisations (NGOs) for their follow-up and support. Especially the Directors and senior managers for devoting their time in providing all the necessary information for this research work.

I am thankful to my family members and also grateful to my friend Luc Vinkx for his unending inspiration and support.

Contents

List of Tables and Figures

Tables

Figures

Abbreviations

AI	Amnesty International
ACSOT	Alliance of Civil Society Organisation of Tigray
AIDS	Acquired Immune Deficiency Syndrome
AIDS FREE	Acquired Immune Deficiency Syndrome – Free
BOPPED	Bureau of Planning and Economic Development
CCM	Comitato Collaborating Medical
CHAI-EPI	Clinton Health Access Initiative - Expanded-Programme-Immunisation
CHAI-MNCH	Clinton Health Access Initiative - Maternal-Neonatal- Child Health
CHAI-PHARM	Clinton Health Access Initiative – Pharmaceutical
CRDA	Christian Relief and Development Association
CSA	Central Statistics Authority
CSO	Civil Society Organisations
DPPB	Disaster Prevention and Preparedness
FDRE	Federal Democratic Republic of Ethiopia
FGAE	Family Guidance Association Ethiopia
FMoH	Federal Ministry of Health
HEW	Health Education Workers
HHOJ	Health Hands of Joy
HIV	Human Immune Deficiency Virus
HMIS	Health Management Information System
INGO	International Non-Governmental Organisations
MFM	Mams for Mams

MOJ	Ministry of Justice
MSI-E	Marie Stops International Ethiopia
NGOs	Non-Governmental Organisations
NHAS	National Health Account Survey
NORAD	Norwegian Agency for Development Cooperation
OSSHD	Organisation for Social Service Health Development
PBS	Protection of Basic Service
REST	Relief Society of Tigray
TRHB	Tigray Regional Health Bureau
Transform PHC	Transform Primary Healthcare
UNDP	United Nations Development Programme
UNICEF	UN International Children's Educational Fund
US	United States
USAID	United States of America International Development
WB	World Bank
WHO	World Health Organisation

1

Introduction

1.1 Introduction

Under this chapter back ground of the study from the objective of the study perspective has been illustrated. Similarly, statement of the problem with the gaps to be addressed, and the aim of the study have described. Besides, objectives of the study, research questions, organisation of the study, the scope and limitation of the study and definition of important terms have briefly been described. Moreover, the research thematic areas with justification have been presented.

1.2 Background of the Study

1.2.1 Overall View of Non-governmental Organisations

The term non-governmental organisations (NGOs) is rooted in the creation of the United Nations in 1945; the title of non-governmental organisations is given to international non-governmental organisations that have acquired consultative status in the activities of the United Nations. To address the problem and how certain writers have been classified by such organisations, they are defined as a third sector which is represented as a non-profit type in anything that you want (Mathew Brown, 2009).

The importance of the evolving non-governmental sector is well explained in the literature on political economy as government and market failure theories. Sociological studies emphasise them as the most important institution improving social integration and being an integral part of a democratic society. The positive attitude towards the non-governmental sector is also predominant in the health sector. The World Health Organisation has acknowledged Non-Governmental Organisations in terms of increasing recognition to complement government programmes and creating an effective people's voice concerning health service requirements and expectations.

1.2.2 Non-Governmental Organisations in Africa

Non-Governmental Organisations make a significant contribution to the developing countries of Africa. According to the Non-Governmental Organisations Sustainability Ranking, the majority of Non-Governmental Organisations in Africa face legal obstacles. Difficulty in obtaining registration is a primary obstacle. In some nations, the Non-Governmental Organisations legislation is obsolete and complex, and the registration process is highly centralised, causing difficulties for Non-Governmental Organisations outside the capital. Non-Governmental Organisations must file at different administrative levels in Angola, Ghana, and Rwanda, which can lead to additional paperwork and delays (USAID, 2009).

In most African countries, especially in Ethiopia, advocacy work is very poor. There is no direct link between Non-Governmental Organisations and policymakers. No coalitions based on issues have been developed and broad-based advocacy programmes have been conducted. Non-Governmental Organisations do not engage in the different levels of government decision-making. Non-Governmental Organisations do not have a favourable situation to lobby the government at different levels to implement or change legislation. However, in Ethiopia, Non-Governmental Organisations are limited by their source of income to activate human rights, democracy, and advocacy to raise 90 percent of their budget from within the country and it is only 10 percent of their total budget that they could raise from abroad (USAID, 2009).

1.2.3 Non-Governmental Organisations in Ethiopia

National and international Non-Governmental Organisations have been active in Ethiopia since the 1960s. Their activities were very restricted during the feudal regime. Thanks to its Marxist-Leninist ideology, the Derg government excluded the majority of Western Non-Governmental Organisations. After the collapse of the "Derg Disaster" in 1991, the majority of Non-Governmental Organisations began to come to work in Ethiopia. Even if most Non-Governmental Organisations have come into existence in the country, there have been no specific laws and regulations governing their registration and operations (Clark, 2004).

The laws and regulations of that time were based on the Ethiopian Civil Code of 1952 and Regulation 321/1959. Nevertheless, this has no longer created a sustainable climate due to the political and other changes that have taken place in Ethiopia. Legislation, which had existed for more than five decades, had become ineffective and was unable to make the most of the country's gains from Non-Governmental Organisations activities. However, some Non-Governmental Organisations have repeatedly asked the government for more up-to-date regulations to allow them to operate smoothly and put an end to resistant procedures and bureaucratic obstacles. The important factor that needed to be taken into account was that, following the collapse of the former military regime and the establishment of the new EPRDF government, the number of foreign Charities increased dramatically due to the introduction of freedom of association in the country (https//:www.chsa.gov.et, 2009). Many Non-Governmental Organisations, especially indigenous, have not internalised democratic cultures. We lack a history of justice and constructive debate and have no media to educate the general public about their acts (g/egziabher, 2002).

1.2.4 Concepts of Healthcare System

According to Oxford English Dictionary, Health, the state of being hale, sound or whole, in the body, mind or soul; in particular, the state of being free from physical illness or pain, or the general condition of the body and mind. Health is a desire for health and happiness as if toasting human beings. Healthcare is a cover for the sick and the wounded to maintain mental and physical health by preventing or treating illness through the services provided by the health profession. The Ethiopian healthcare system is characterised by extreme long-term financial and human resource deficits, poor healthcare facilities and decades of lack of a strong national health policy. (Richard G. & Wamai, 2004) Ethiopia also has one of the worst health outcomes in the world. Mortality and maternal mortality rates are very high 66 per 1000 live births and 850 per 100,000 live births, respectively.

The health sector policy of Ethiopia has different and diverse stakeholders, both within and outside of the health sector. For certain cases, the assignment of various tasks to stakeholders is not well defined due to overlapping roles. As seen for the table, Non-Governmental Organisations are funding curative and preventive services. We also have curative, preventive and drug-related services. Many Non-Governmental Organisations are not domestic, far removed from many social and cultural aspects of society, and many Non-Governmental Organisations tend to retain institutional and personal interests rather than the broader beneficiary (Zewdie & Pausewan, 2002).

1.2.5 The Healthcare Service in Ethiopia

State profile and health policy growth like many other countries in sub-Saharan Africa, Ethiopia is a state with diverse cultures, customs, and history. Despite its ancient civilisations and being the only other country on the continent not colonised as well as one of the oldest territorially dependent nations in the world, Ethiopia is currently one of the least developed countries in the world. In contrast, for example, even though Ethiopia has more than twice the population of neighbouring Kenya, its healthcare system is about one-third of Kenya's population in terms of services and resources. It is also the third most populous country in Africa with a population of about 112 million. Eighty-two percent of the population live on less than a dollar a day, 44 percent live below the national poverty line (Richard G. & Wamai, 2009).

Hence in line to these theoretical concepts the researcher deals on this study to assess and identify the gaps in the practices and challenges of the Non-Governmental Organisations in providing healthcare service in the selected study in Tigray Regional State, Northern Ethiopia.

1.3 Statement of the Problem

Over the last few decades, Ethiopia has seen an increase in the number of Non-Governmental Organisations due to a combination of factors. Four hundred Non-Governmental Organisations in Ethiopia are managing health projects or projects that potentially contribute to lessening major public health problems in the country. The majority of Non-Governmental Organisationswork in the regional states of Ethiopia. Non-Governmental Organisations are active in the provision of health services, rehabilitation and extension of health services, human resource development, pharmaceutical services, and improvement of the health and information systems, organisational analysis, IEC and healthcare financing. Non-Governmental Organisations are providing curative, preventive and rehabilitative health services.

They manage first and second level health unit's health offices, clinics, health centers and hospitals in the country's healthcare system. Ethiopia ratified the policy of the health sector and subsequently launched a 20-year Health Sector Development Programme (HSDP). The HSDP responds to a number of issues identified in the coverage and quality of health services. It is divided into four consecutive five-year plans and the first and second stages span the period 1997-2002 and the period 2002-2005. The priorities for these periods are: (a) Increase access and availability of healthcare along with utilisation; (b) Enhance quality of service through training and increased delivery of the required inputs; and (c) Strengthen management of health services at the federal and regional levels. One of the methods used to accomplish these goals is to promote the participation of the private sector and Non-Governmental Organisations, by creating conducive environment. When part of the national healthcare reform, the former six-tier system was replaced by a four-tier system (Charity & Society Agency, 2017).

According to the Ethiopia Health Strategy, the Primary Healthcare Unit (PHCU) has one health center and five satellite health posts first level care provider in the health service delivery of the country. The Ethiopian Government is increasingly interested in working with non-governmental organisations, and Non-Governmental Organisations are also emerging as new institutional actors in the socio-economic development of Ethiopia. To date, different activities / strategies and mechanisms are being used to strengthen GO-NGO collaboration in the health sector at regional level. Non-Governmental Organisations participate in the HSDP of Ethiopia through development of health infrastructure, delivery of health services, development of human resources, capacity building of health facilities, prevention of communicable diseases, supply of essential drugs and emergency nutritional supplements and therapeutic food intervention in food crisis situations. Charity organisations previously focused on relief and support, but currently the majority of charities are active in the field of sustainable development. Non-Governmental Organisations are working on microfinance, capacity building and self-reliance. The researcher also agrees that these three elements are very important. According to (Cheston S. & Kuhn L., 2002), microfinance is one of the most common forms of economic empowerment for women, which provides credit for poor women who are usually excluded from formal credit institutions. Attention to poverty reduction for women in poor households is necessary if the Millennium Development Goals to reduce poverty are to be achieved. Not only are women the majority of poor people, but they are likely to invest surpluses in healthcare, better education, school fees and other household needs, resulting in a decrease in child and household poverty Measurements in terms of nutrition, consumption and well-being (Cheston S. & Kuhn L., 2002).

The above studies had been conducted in Ethiopia that reveals the issues of the capacity-builders to help the community develop resources, raise awareness, motivate project participation and, improve the quality of community life, microfinance, capacity building and self-reliance.

However, this study did not address in the practice and challenges of Non-Governmental Organisations in supporting healthcare service in Tigray Regional State, Northern Ethiopia. Therefore, the researcher was intended to conduct the research in the study area.

1.3.1 Research Gap

The aim of this study is to find out the gap on practice and challenge of healthcare service supported by NGOs they have been engage in the healthcare service development programme for quite sometimes so in respect to the length of period that they have been in operation in the programme the organisations, they are expected to bring about improvement which is mainly solve problem and not forming competitive business.

Therefore, it is important to ask what the existing practice and challenges looks like in these Non-Governmental Organisations and also assess the healthcare service support that are being used by these Non-Governmental Organisations to ensure their transparency and accountability and enhance their project performance. Accordingly, the study has addressed the following research objectives and questions.

1.4 Objectives of the Study

In this study there are two types of objectives. These are the general objective, and the specific objectives. To highlight it, the purpose of this study is to assess and identify the gaps in the practices and challenges of the Non-Governmental Organisations in supporting healthcare service in the selected study area Tigray Region, Northern Ethiopia, 2020.

1.4.1 General Objectives

The general objective of the study is assessing the practices and challenges of non-governmental organisations in supporting healthcare service.

1.4.2 Specific Objectives

1. To assess the practices of non-governmental organisations in supporting the healthcare services.
2. To identify the major challenges faced by non-governmental organisations in supporting healthcare services.

1.4.3 Research Questions

1. What are the practices of Non-Governmental Organisations in supporting the healthcare services?
2. What are the challenges faced by Non-Governmental Organisations in supporting the healthcare services?

1.5 Significance of the Study

The practice of services supports by Non-Governmental Organisations in the healthcare service and the overall challenges faced during the implementation time. Studies should enhance our awareness of the practice that Non-Governmental Organisations play in particular in supporting and enhancing the livelihoods of society in general. The study will improve policymakers and health practitioners by paying due attention to the quality of healthcare services and the practice of Non-Governmental Organisations. The research explores the magnitude of the contribution made by Non-Governmental Organisations to the chosen healthcare sector and its relation to society.

The study was discussed the practice and challenges of non-governmental organisations in supporting healthcare services and their contribution to the progress and strategy of achieving the goals of the healthcare system. Besides, the development of this research identifies the key issue facing Non-Governmental Organisations when they are engaged in healthcare and provide practical solutions to these problems. The results of this study will provide information for a wide range of users, such as health policymakers, academics, and Non-Governmental Organisations for themselves. Specifically, healthcare supporters could use the findings of this study to enhance the engagement of Non-Governmental Organisations in all activities of community healthcare. Therefore, this research was undertaken to generate and add some evidence-based information to existing knowledge of Non-Governmental Organisations practice on the factors that contribute to health system management policy and the sustainable development of the public healthcare service sector as a whole. This study was a baseline to the closed relation with the government and Non-Governmental Organisations and with other partners during implementation and there should be a mutual understanding among the organisations to implement the laws and policies of healthcare service. This study will give the findings and recommendations of the study for the future use to the Policymakers, implementers, users, to the community or beneficiaries, and this study can serve as reference for other researchers those who can make farther investigation in the target area.

1.6 Scope of the Study

Thematically or in content the scope of this study focuses on the practices and challenges of Non-Governmental Organisations; at the exploratory level. Geographically it focuses on Non-Governmental Organisations supporting the healthcare sector in Tigray Regional State, Northern Ethiopia. The study considers 35 NGOs those who participate in the selected study area, the government leaders and officers. The study was restricted only in the Tigray region healthcare sector and it does not include the general situation of other governmental sectors in the study area.

1.6.1 Geographical and Respondent Scope

The study was carried out in Non-Governmental Organisations that are under the support of the healthcare service in Tigray

Regional State. The target population involved in the healthcare service of the surveyed 120 leaders and workers of 35 Non-Governmental Organisations in Tigray.

1.6.2 Content Scope

The study assessed the practice and challenge of Non-Governmental Organisations in supporting healthcare service in Tigray Regional State, Tigray.

1.7 Description of the Study

Tigray Regional is the northernmost of the nine regions of Ethiopia, with a rich history and culture. It is the source of Geez Field (Alphabet), Christianity, and Islam in Ethiopia. It is the land of Saint Yared who was known for his religious songs and melodies, Axum and its obelisk, Yeha and Wuqro, Al Negashi, and dauntless Emperors such as: Ezana, Kaleb, Yohannes and other many more.Tigray is bordered by Eritrea to the North, Sudan to the West, the Afar Region to the East, and the Amhara Region to the South and Southwest. The total area of the Region is about 54,569.25 km^2 with population of 5,510,511 where (Male 2,716,923 and Female 2,793,588), and its capital city is Mekelle. The region is administratively divided in to 7 Zones including one special zone, Mekelle. It has 52 woredas (District) (34 Rural and 18 Urban) and 814 Kebelles or Tabiyas (722 Rural and 92 Urban). Countries of erosion, deforestation, and overgrasing have left the region with dry and treeless plains, hills, and plateaus. Nevertheless, Tigray has an amasing landscape with the Tekeze Gorge at 550 meters above sea level and the mountains like Kisad Gudo peaking at 3935 meters. Cliff ledges and precipices are natural attractions of the Region. Tigray's natural scenery is classified as central highlands, the western lowland, and eastern escarpments. The climate of the region is characterised as 39 percent kola, (semi-arid), 49 percent weina dega (warm temperate), and 12 percent dega (temperate). The annual regional rainfall ranges from 450 to 980 millimeters.

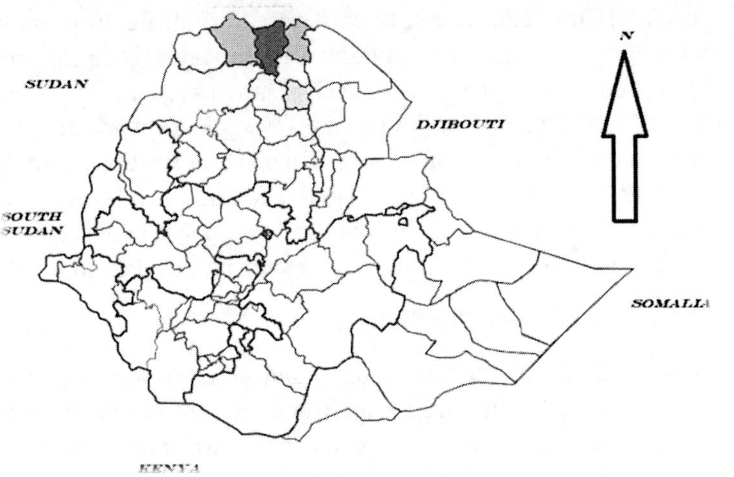

Fig. 1.1: Map of the study area Ethiopia – Tigray

Source: Tigray Regional Health Bureau HMIS.

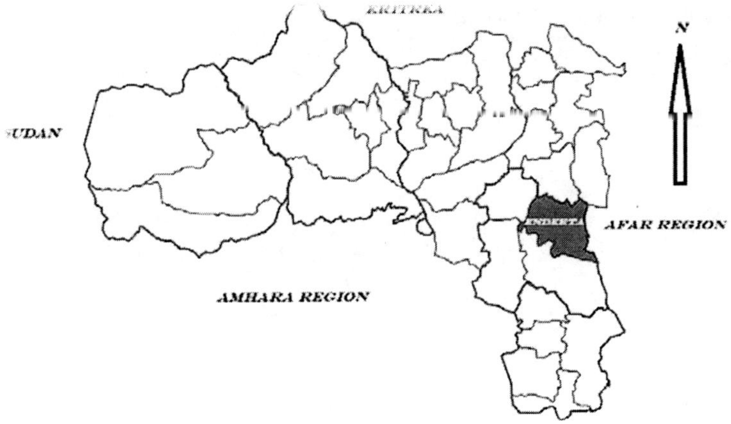

Fig. 1.2: Map of study area Tigray

Source: Tigray Regional Health Bureau HMIS.

1.8 Limitations of the Study

This study was conducted in the Tigray Regional States, the Northern Ethiopia. The assessment on the practice and challenges of Non-Governmental Organisations in supporting the healthcare service in the region. Here, threats were very difficult to assess and to get data from the concerned bodies, non-governmental organisations due to the situational Corona virus (covid-19) disease was very difficult in facilitating the researcher's work and, the concerned organisations an openness to give information about the research. The reason that they rise is because of the security of the head office do not have willing to give response to the research report. These were difficult to the expected collect data smoothly.

1.9 Organisation of the Study

After finalising this thesis, the organisation of this study will have five chapters with well-established sections in each chapter. Chapter one is the introduction part, chapter two contains a review of related literatures. Chapter three involves the methodology and discussion part. Chapter four includes analysing of data, presentation and interpretation of the study. The final chapter is chapter five and it contains a summary of the major findings, conclusions, and recommendations.

2

Literature Reviews

2.1 Introduction

In the twenty-first century, non-governmental organisations (NGOs) are a significant part of the international system as the world becomes increasingly globalised and the problems of lesser-developed nations become more apparent through the application of foreign policy. By the World Bank definition, Non-Governmental Organisations are defined as "private organisations that pursue activities to relieve the suffering, promote the interests of the poor, protect the environment, provide basic social services, or undertake community development."[1] Especially with regards to non-profits, the image that is often perceived by the majority of people is that these organisations, because of their charitable nature, are autonomous, credible, "do-good" institutions free from politics or corruption. Unfortunately, a closer inspection of the finances of these organisations reveals that these institutions are more significantly linked to government and private donor agendas than their name would inherently lead one to believe. The majority of Non-Governmental Organisations financing can be characterised by two different relationships: one between the Non-Governmental Organisations and the private investor, and the second between the Non-Governmental Organisations and a government (which can be either a host government or a foreign one). Non-Governmental Organisations and donor relations can further be analysed to include demand-led and supply-led contracts. In a demand-led situation, Non-Governmental Organisations are in control of the projects and their implementation, while donors have a small voice when determining which of the presented options to fund. This scenario is ideal for Non-Governmental Organisations, as they retain the most in control of their institution and the progress that is made. However, should the situation be supply-led, which is the case more often than not, then donors are in charge of creating and implementing the programmes of the organisation. This supply-led scenario is dangerous for Non-Governmental Organisations because it is when they are most reliant on a single donor's funds, and have little say in the activities of their own organisation. By giving donors excessive power, Non-Governmental Organisations sacrifice autonomy, credibility, and in some cases their core mission and values. The resulting situation is one in which donors can easily manipulate the organisation to their own desires and agendas. These organisations have limited options when it comes to reacting to a donor change in objectives, of the three: exit, voice, and adjustment, they more often adjust to the donor demands, ultimately resulting in mission creep.

The second major relationship that increases Non-Governmental Organisations' vulnerability to funding manipulation is with the government, either the host or a foreign state. Non-Governmental Organisations and governments can contradict one another, and an unhealthy relationship of mistrust can result in serious obstacles in the organisation's effectiveness and ability to actually assist citizens in its mission. The most efficient way for governments to control Non-Governmental Organisations is by controlling their funding resources. Countries such as Russia and Egypt have implemented laws which restrict Non-Governmental Organisations' ability to receive international funding for fear of outside government manipulation and infiltration into the host government. At the risk of being charged with treason, most organisations in these nations are now unable to deliver services and aid to the beneficiaries of their programmes and are forced to rely on host government funds to finance operations. Over reliance on government funding is another characteristic which causes Non-Governmental Organisations to become more vulnerable to manipulation. Organisations which are closely involved with government projects, missions, and objectives are more likely to acquiesce to behaviours that would otherwise be intolerable. Additionally, the number of advocacy Non-Governmental Organisations drops considerably when they are dependent on government funding, which affects the overall dynamic of the sector within a country. Overall, while government funding is more stable than private donor funds, the conflict of interests as Non-Governmental Organisations try to balance the accountability to their investors and their beneficiaries is a slippery slope which all too often leads to funds manipulation.

Non-Governmental Organisations have the ability to counteract these hazards to their autonomy and credibility through adjustments in three main aspects of their organisation: finance, individual, and international. Firstly, Non-Governmental Organisations can better counteract funding manipulation by diversifying their resources. If they can avoid dependence on a single donor or government, then they are more likely to have the option to walk away rather than adjust to demands from either entity. This also lessens the financial risk and burden as donors are constantly fluctuating their core subject and diversification allows an organisation to have more fluidity in their sources. Non-Governmental Organisations can also take individual measures to avoid funding manipulation through creating relationships with donors in order to have a space to voice their opinion, being committed to their mission above finances, and investing in their own organisation. These proactive measures increase the strength and commitment of the institution to their original purpose and decrease the chances of goal displacement. Finally, on the international level, donors can have more accountability for the negative consequences of their conditional lending and fund long term projects that benefit the organisation and host country as a whole. Donors can increase demand-led scenarios and decrease the pressure on Non-Governmental Organisations to prioritise them above the beneficiaries.

This thesis intends to assess the practice and challenges of Non-Governmental Organisations on governmental health services centers. Hypothesise that smaller to Medium-size organisations are vulnerable because they have smaller boards and therefore have greater disadvantages when it comes to board resources and performance; these disadvantages include less access to financial resources which in turn leads to supply-led contracts. Market competition is another variable due to its influence on the degree to which Non-Governmental Organisations has to outperform other organisations and what funding options are therefore available to the Non-Governmental Organisations. I also hypothesise that high market competition among Non-Governmental Organisations combined with low market competition among donors creates a toxic combination of supply-led contracts. Additionally, I hypothesise that Non-Governmental Organisations with targeted funding is weaker because it creates donor dependence and limits the Non-Governmental Organisations available reactions to donor demands, which again implies a supply-led contract. All three hypotheses have the same result of supply led contracts, and these supply-led contracts perpetuate funding manipulation by creating a vulnerability to intuitional isomorphism by the donor's excessive power and control over the organisation.

In Ethiopia the History of Non-Government Organisations traces its origin back to the establishment of self-help organisations like Debo, Idir and Ikub. These are traditionally established institutions and they facilitate mutual support among their members of the community. In the countryside of Ethiopia farmers support each other and specially support widows and peoples in old age during farming and harvest seasons by the collaboration called Debo. The other association, Idir serves as an institution that provides insurance and support for its members during emergency and death. In addition to that according their constitution different Idirs are involved in several other activities. Ikub serves as a saving institution which provides lump sum of money collected from its member based on lots casting and some other arrangements (Clark, 2000).

In 1960 both foreign and local Non-Governmental Organisations were established when these self-help groups could no longer suffice to support the needy of the country. The development department of Ethiopian Evangelical Church Mekane Yesus (EECMY) is the first official religious local Non-Governmental Organisations formally established in the 1960s to coordinate education, medical and rural development programmes.

The first secular Non-Governmental Organisations as we know them today that were established in the country were the Ethiopian Red Cross and Swedish save the children following this and the famine of 1973 and later of 1984 the number of Non-Governmental Organisations increased and these were mostly international. As a matter of fact, neither the feudal dynasty nor the Dergue regime were not prepared to address the famine problem of 1970s and 1980s but Non-Governmental Organisations were instrumentals in preventing greater loss of life in both catastrophic episodes. Two decades ago, the Ethiopian famine, which witnessed by the world was a cause for the death of more than one million people and many more were suffering. It left a tragic effect in the history of the country.

Later on, with the change in government in 1990 a more conducive environment was established further encouraging the growth of Non-Governmental Organisations in Ethiopia. This time as their numbers increased more local Non-Governmental Organisations flourished. Since then the number of Non-Governmental Organisations were very few and structurally, they very week. During the feudal regime in Ethiopia Non-Governmental Organisations has no considerable activity. Even if there were few Non-Governmental Organisations, they were involved in relief activities. During the Dergue regime due to the Marxist-Leninist indoctrination philosophy, Non-Governmental Organisations had no freedom to operate in the country and were seen suspiciously and even most Non-Governmental Organisations were forced to leave the country.

2.2 Concepts of Non-Governmental Organisations

Non-governmental organisations (NGOs) usually have a very distinctive feature as private institutions serving public purposes. These are known by various names around the world, such as

- non-profit organisations;
- third-sector organisations;
- voluntary organisations;
- community-based organisations;
- charitable organisations, and so on.

Though their nature and focus of activities have changed over time, they have gained prominence in a wide spectrum of activities cutting across economic, social, cultural and scientific domains. Nowadays, the nongovernmental sector is recognised as a major social and economic force in almost all countries (Rajeev, 2016). In the broader definitions, Non-Governmental Organisations are "associations formed within civil society bringing together individuals who share common purpose" (Pluto, 1996).

According to (GTZ, 2011), in the Ethiopian context, Non-Governmental Organisations is an organisation that meets the following requirements: Non-Governmental Organisations are voluntary in their genesis; Non-Governmental Organisations engage in relief, service delivery, advocacy or development activities; Non-Governmental Organisations are non-profit or self-serving organisations working to serve the disadvantaged groups of the society; Non-Governmental Organisations are non-political; Non-Governmental Organisations have no permanent programme interest or geographical context; Non-Governmental Organisations refers to both indigenous and international non-governmental organisations. Non-Governmental Organisations have very special characteristics, as they are usually private institutions that serve the public. Non-Governmental Organisations around the world are regularly referred to under different names, such as non-profit organisations, third-party organisations, voluntary organisations, community-based organisations, charities and the like. Although their nature and the focus of their activities have changed over time, they have gained widespread access to activities such as economic, social, cultural and scientific fields. Nowadays, the non-governmental sector is considered to have social and economic power in almost every country.

The importance and visibility of Non-Governmental Organisations are closely related to the Ethiopian famines. Ethiopia experienced two crippling famines in 1973/74 and 1984/85, causing forced mass migration and a major loss of life and wealth. These famines resulted in a dramatic increase in the number of NGOs operating in the country (Kassa, 2015).

Non-Government organisations most of the time referred to as Civil Society Organisations (CSOs) are organisations that are established to serve the public voluntarily and most often established as not for profit. As it's evident from the name Non-Government Organisation implies any organisation which does not include government or government-appointed officials in its membership. Non-Governmental Organisations are one of the main actors in the development process. When Non-Governmental Organisations play their role properly, they are a strong supporting arm to the government. It is hoped that they will play an active role in poverty reduction and sustainable development.

The term third sector is granted to Non-Governmental Organisations because the first sector is the government sector and the second sector is the private sector and Non-Governmental Organisations are the third sector (Lewis, Davis & Kanji, 2009). The Non-Governmental Organisations have the following five key characteristics; it is formal, that is, the organisation is institutionalised in that it has regular meetings, office holders and some organisational continuity.

2.2.1 Types of Non-Governmental Organisations

Non-Governmental Organisations (NGOs) can be categorised into different types based on their different factors, such as ideology or level of cooperation. Non-Governmental Organisations category by orientation can be grouped into charitable orientation; service orientation; participatory orientation; and empowerment of orientation. The Non-Governmental Organisations may be divided into Community-based organisations, the City-Wide Organisation, regional Non-Governmental Organisations and the International Non-Governmental Organisations. Non-governmental organisations are a heterogeneous group and work in different areas with a wide range of work. We also use different terminology to refer to these Non-Governmental Organisations including private voluntary organisations, civil society, the independent sector, self-help organisations and grassroots organisations, the voluntary sector, transitional social movement organisations and non-state actors (Sunshant, 2010).

The global community of Non-Governmental Organisations encompasses a wide range of organisations, which can usually be categorised into three basic types; (a) Humanitarian aid, both emergency response and development. (b) Advocacy groups right to advocate for groups such as women, children, disabled people, and disadvantaged groups in society. (c) Faith-based groups are humanitarian groups formed based on faith principles. Missionary aid groups aim to "spread the word" through charitable access to those in need of religious instruction. Faith-based charities have the strength from faith-based teachings to carry out charitable activities.

According to the World Health Organisation (WHO), each national health system should be directed to achieve three overall goals: good health, responsiveness to the expectations of the population, and fairness of financial contribution Progress towards them depend crucially on how well the systems execute four vital functions. These include the provision of services, production of capital, funding, and stewardship. Comparing the way these functions are carried out provides a basis for understanding performance variations over time and among countries (UNICEF, 2017b).

Health system includes all the activities with the purpose to promote, restore and maintain health. It means that the health system is the complex of interrelated elements that contribute to health in homes, educational institutions, workplaces, public places, and communities, as well as in physical and psychosocial climate, wellbeing and related fields. The health system is typically structured at different levels, beginning at the most peripheral level, also known as the community level or the primary level of healthcare, and progressing from the intermediate level (district, national or provincial) to the central level. The intermediate and central levels deal with those aspects of the healthcare system that provide increasingly more complicated and advanced care and support. The infrastructure of the health system includes services, facilities, institutions or establishments, organisations and those that operate them for the delivery of a variety of health services and programmes. They provide individuals, families, and communities with healthcare that consists of a combination of promoted, protective, preventive, diagnostic, curative and rehabilitative measures.

In most African countries, especially in Ethiopia, support work is very poor. There is no direct link between Non-Governmental Organisations and policymakers. No coalitions based on issues have been developed and broad-based advocacy programmes have been conducted. Non-Governmental Organisations do not engage in the different levels of government decision-making. Non-Governmental Organisations do not have a favourable situation to lobby the government at different levels to implement or change legislation. However, in Ethiopia, Non-Governmental Organisations are limited by their source of income to activate human rights, democracy, and advocacy to raise 90 percent of their budget from within the country and it is only 10 percent of their total budget that they could earn from abroad (UNICEF, 2017b).

Ethiopia, like most developing countries, is struggling with insufficient resources to meet the basic health needs of its rapidly growing and overwhelmingly young population, in the face of severe poverty, the cycle of natural disasters, the AIDS epidemic, and persistent conflicts. The Government of Ethiopia is the country's leading western healthcare provider. Due to the country's past political philosophy and socio-economic situations, there is minimal involvement of Non-Governmental Organisations and the private sector in the delivery of services, even though voluntary, church-based and missionary organisations have been leaders in the implementation of modern medical services in Ethiopia. The first health institution in Ethiopia was founded and operated by the Russian Red Cross Medical Team during the reign of Emperor Menelik II. Church-based organisations and missionaries were significant healthcare providers in the country in the first quarter of the twentieth century. Marginalised health issues such as leprosy, physical/mental disability, birth-related fistula, post-abortion treatment, family planning services, and HIV /AIDS are some of the concerns of the Non-Governmental Organisations in Ethiopia (https//:www.chsa.gov.et, 2009). Over the last half-century, the involvement of non-governmental and voluntary groups in the health sector has gradually increased. The 1997 assessment shows that 146 health facilities are managed by this sector. The mid-term HSDP review reports that 10 percent of the health -care is provided by the Non-Governmental sector (https//:www.chsa.gov.et, 2009). Some groups of Civil Society Organisations (CSOs) were active in Ethiopia before the existence of "Non-Governmental Organisations". Traditional self-help programmes were the first organisations in Ethiopia to be identified as NGOs. Such self-help organisations, such as "Iddirs" and "Mahbers," have been there for years, bringing depth to the civil society landscape in Ethiopia (Charity & Society Agency, 2017).

In 1960, both foreign and local Non-Governmental Organisations were set up when these self-help organisations could no longer be sufficient to support the country's poor. The first Non-Governmental Organisations known today to have been founded in the country were the Ethiopian Red Cross and the Swedish Children's Save. Following this and the famine of 1973 and later in 1984, the number of Non-Governmental Organisations increased, most of them internationally. Later on, with the change of government in 1990, a more favourable climate was created to further encourage the growth of Non-Governmental Organisations in Ethiopia. Some 3,822 Non-Governmental Organisations have been registered in Ethiopia for more than half a century from the 1950s to 2009 to operate in different areas. Since its formation in 2009, the new Charities and Societies Agency has re-registered 739 national and international Non-Governmental Organisations (Charity & Society Agency, 2017). This means that almost 40 percent of the 3822 Non-Governmental Organisations registered before the new Proclamation was issued. More than 2,000 Non-Governmental Organisations have been licenced under Proclamation No. 621/2009. Of these, more than 1,600 are growth and welfare-related domestic and foreign charities. As of 09 December 2014, more than 500 Non-Governmental Organisations have been registered and licenced by the Agency to work on environmental protection. Also, the Agency has registered close to 98 Ethiopian organisations and societies that have the right to work on human rights and conflict resolution (Charity & Society Agency, 2017).

According to the (Christian Relief & Development Association, 2014), the development of Non-Governmental Organisations in Ethiopia can be divided into three phases. The first step was the complete participation of the sector in relief and humanitarian work.

Non-governmental organisations have been active during the Ethiopian human rights crisis. According to the Marxist-Leninist Creed, during the Dergue regime, Non-Governmental Organisations were not free to operate in the country and were even suspicious, and many Non-Governmental Organisations were forced to leave the country. According to Proclamation 621/2009, there is a dichotomy between human rights and development. This is impossible, according to the critics. Growth and human rights are very interrelated issues. Many factors lead to underdevelopment in developing countries like ours. Development activities have their contribution to socio-economic rights. Most African countries have gone through internal and external conflicts that have been attributed to their underdevelopment.

Based on one source citing a household welfare survey on health utilisation, 3.3 percent of respondents reported using Non-Governmental Organisations services. The second National Health Account reported that in 2000 the Ethiopian health Non-Governmental Organisations community-contributed 10 percent of the national health expenditure. A larger portion of fees paid for health services is spent in non-MOH facilities and, as one study found, cost-recovery in Non-Governmental Organisations facilities is 70 percent (Hellinger, 1987b).

Although Non-Governmental Organisations are expected to report their activities to the regional health authorities where they work, the reporting appears to be only haphazard. This makes accurate data hard to find. Reported data are coded and entered into the national health management information system (HMIS), where it becomes difficult to disaggregate. Like other civil society organisations, there is no common agreement among Non-Governmental Organisations on global definitions. Non-Governmental Organisations are more broadly defined as "associations established within civil society that bring together individuals who share a common interest" (Turner & Hulme, 2008).

2.3 Theoretical Literatures

The key role and practice of Non-Governmental Organisations in the health sector is the capacity to deliver local health services directly. In many cases, these distributions can be seen as an extension of the business. Religious-affiliated hospitals have a particularly large market share in Africa. Non-Governmental Organisations may also have a comparative advantage when the operation serves specialised public goods, requires specialised knowledge and is difficult to reach. In some cases, Non-

Governmental Organisations play a role in community organising around health issues. We will help coordinate groups to identify and respond to health needs (Henwood, Nicholson, 2005).

This is common in countries with poor public health systems, where both people and donors are seeking alternative delivery mechanisms. The expansion of health-related Non-Governmental Organisations in Haiti, funded by the United States Agency for International Development (USAID) and other donors, is a case in point. Most notably those on the margins of society who may or may not be supported by public and private-sector providers. Such communities include indigenous peoples, women in patriarchal cultures, sex workers and slum dwellers. Examples of Non-Governmental Organisations that respond effectively to the needs of these communities include Prosalud in Bolivia, Building Resources in all countries, (BRAC) in Bangladesh, Mexfam in Mexico, and Partners for Health in Haiti and Peru. Other notable examples are the provision of health insurance and key health services by the Self-Employed Women's Association (SEWA) in India to its members, and the African Nutrition Programme to the most isolated people in Uganda and Burundi (Henwood, Nicholson, 2005).

2.3.1 The Practice of Non-Governmental Organisations

Health inequities are caused by some determinants, including the use or access to healthcare facilities. Work addressing these issues involves a cross-sectional approach involving cross-disciplinary teams and methodologies. Building trans-disciplinary teams require the commitment of the research community to seek out colleagues from other disciplines, funding agencies to appreciate innovative initiatives, the broader community as partners and contributors, and the policy arena to develop intersectional policy strategies and programmes that may well be directed outside the ministries of health. Nonetheless, operating outside the government as a whole may well be a viable and effective policy (UNICEF, 2017a).

Non-Governmental Organisations have very special characteristics, as they are usually private institutions that serve the public. Non-Governmental Organisations around the world are regularly referred to under different names, such as non-profit organisations, third-party organisations, voluntary organisations, community-based organisations, charities and the like. Although their nature and the focus of their activities have changed over time, they have gained widespread access to activities such as economic, social, cultural and scientific fields. Nowadays, the non-governmental sector is considered to have social and economic power in almost every country. In the health sector, the World Health Organisation has agreed to support Non-Governmental Organisations in the implementation of government programmes and the promotion of active human voices in the area of health service needs and expectations. In creating a collaborative system to improve performance in the health sector, most countries around the world have expanded the opportunity to participate in the provision of health services (Anurag Priyadarshee, 2010).

The context of health reforms and decentralisation Ethiopia is one of the least developed countries in the world with low development indicators even by sub-Saharan Africa standards. Eighty-five percent of the country's population of 70 million lives in rural areas, 44 percent living below the national poverty line (the Federal Democratic Republic of Ethiopia (Anurag Priyadarshee, 2010). National average health coverage is 64 percent but utilisation per capita is only 0.36 Federal Ministry of Health (Anurag Priyadarshee, 2010). Following over 20 years of dictatorship under the Dergue regime, in the early 1990s, a new democratic government took power and set a new environment for health policy. The new Constitution set a federal system of government comprising nine autonomous largely ethnically distinct regions and two administrative councils, which were further sub-divided into sixty-two zones and 523 woredas (districts) (Hellinger, 1987b). In 1993 the government published the first health policy in 50 years setting the vision for developing the healthcare sector for the next 20 years (Hellinger, 1987a). Some of the aspects of this policy focus on radical reforms in the system including decentralisation, expanding the primary healthcare system and encouraging partnerships and the participation of private and Non-Governmental Organisations actors. To translate the policy for implementation the first Health Sector Development Programme (HSDP-I) was launched in 1997/98.

2.3.2 Challenges of Non-Governmental Organisations

Non-Governmental Organisations (NGOs) are faced with challenges such as complex requirements and expectations; Non-Governmental Organisations are highly dependent on the flow of resources from external providers. This dependency can create a situation in which donors have power over the Non-Governmental Organisations, the interests of the funding agency conflict with the interests of the organisation, Non-Governmental Organisations are left with two options: seek funding from other sources, or make the necessary changes to obtain funding reference was made to why Family Health International (FHI) was not ablc to secure funding from donors due to conflict of the interests. Non-Governmental Organisations with higher levels of dependency may be forced to make these changes to ensure their survival. Lack of proper coordination, undermining of the county health department, poor communication and lack of transparency were some of the issues reported during the research. Bureaucracy in the government departments also affects the delivery of the health services and further frustrates the work of Non-Governmental Organisations in the health sector.

Non-Governmental Organisations make a significant contribution to the developing countries of Africa. According to the 2009 USAID Non-Governmental Organisations Sustainability Ranking, the majority of Non-Governmental Organisations in Africa face legal obstacles. Difficulty in obtaining registration is a primary obstacle. In some nations, the Non-Governmental Organisations legislation is obsolete and complex, and the registration process is highly centralised, causing difficulties for Non-Governmental Organisations outside the capital. Non-Governmental Organisations must file at different administrative levels in Angola, Ghana, and Rwanda, which can lead to additional paperwork and delays (USAID, 2017).

Another challenge is any countries encroaching on legal provisions restrict the ability of Non-Governmental Organisations to support themselves financially. Non-Governmental Organisations in Burundi, for instance, do not benefit from tax exemptions; even in countries that offer tax exemptions or other financial incentives to Non-Governmental Organisations, such as the DRC and Guinea, processes are often so complex that few Non-Governmental Organisations can take advantage of them. There are no fiscal incentives in Sierra Leone to encourage individual and corporate donors to donate to Non-Governmental Organisations. Bureaucratic conditions in Mali disqualify Non-Governmental Organisations from participating in certain government tenders and Non-Governmental Organisations legislation that imposes unnecessary limits, such as in Ethiopia, where Non-Governmental Organisations receiving foreign funding are prevented from working on topics deemed to be politically sensitive (USAID, 2009).

In some countries, such as the DRC and Senegal, Non-Governmental Organisations have recognised the need for more inclusive legislation and are pursuing initiatives to improve it, but this is not a top priority for Non-Governmental Organisations in other countries such as Nigeria. In Ghana, Non-Governmental Organisations have opposed a proposed Non-Governmental Organisations law that they claim could limit their growth and activities (USAID, 2009). In the past, the governance system has given little room for the development of a powerful and vibrant civil society over Ethiopia. The hierarchical and autocratic nature of governance contributed significantly to the small and emerging civil society in general and the poor disintegrated the Non-Governmental Organisations sector in particular in the country (World Bank, 2000). The year 1991 was considered more positive about the growth of a stable civil society in Ethiopia. Since that time, it has not been questioned that more civil society has been created as a result of a relatively improved political environment.

External Challenges

Government attitude: Strong, vibrant and independent institutions have been seen as a threat by the present government and have been categorised as part of the opposition and are working to undermine its power bases (Desalegn, 2008). There has been a marked improvement in the relationship between Non-Governmental Organisations and the state immediately after the war with Eritrea, due to the government's desire to win support for civil society after the war; however, the government has no interest and appetite in seeing Non-Governmental Organisations and other civil society sectors as real development partner.

Bureaucracy: Long and cumbersome procedures for registration, strict reporting requirements and growing lack of transparency on the part of government executive bodies are exacerbating the ever-volatile relationship between the Government and Non-Governmental Organisations (Campbell, 1996).

Pro-government Non-Governmental Organisations (NGOs): The government actively funds its own party-controlled, parallel civil society groups, such as local indigenous Non-Governmental Organisations, women's organisations, youth councils, and trade unions. It confirms the fear in the voluntary sector that the state does not trust and may plan to replace independent civil society groups in the future (Zewdie & Pausewan, 2002).

Participation: Major decisions affecting civil society itself are made at the national and federal level without the involvement of civil society representatives. A simple case in point is that officials in the Ministry of Justice responsible for drafting new legislation governing Non-Governmental Organisations operations have not been able to include the Non-Governmental Organisations sector in the preparatory effort (CRDA, 2006a).The report of the Norwegian Agency for Development Cooperation (NORAD) on the Capacity Building Programme in Ethiopia (2005) stated that the Ethiopian Government is considerably more restrictive in terms of the space it offers to international and national Non-

Governmental Organisations than the Sri Lankan State (Norad, 2005).

Rules and regulations: It is the State that lays down the laws, the legislation regulating the obligations of civil society and the rules are ambiguous, unrealistic and subject to arbitrary interpretation by the regulatory authorities (CRDA, 2006b). With the idea systematic enforcement of the law, contrary to the provisions of their parent legislation, restricted freedom of association, violated the fundamental provisions of the constitutions and international human rights treaties ratified by Ethiopia. In addition to the above instances, it is possible to list more similar challenges. Nevertheless, what has been said so far can demonstrate how hostile the working environment is to non-governmental organisations in particular and the involvement of civil society in general? It is important to mention here that the structural constraints are the main bottlenecks that are the most difficult to overcome and are responsible for restricting the wider participation of non-governmental organisations (CRDA, 2006a).

Internal Challenges

Capacity limitation: There is a significant limitation of the capacity of indigenous Non-Governmental Organisations. Limiting human resources and budget constraints are key features of local Non-Governmental Organisations. The lack of access to resources, physical assets, and human capital is characteristic of Ethiopian Non-Governmental Organisations.

Weak private sector: In Ethiopia, the private sector is so weak and fragile as to become internal sources of funding for Non-Governmental Organisations, as is the case in many other countries. The private sector is so weak as a result of unfriendly policy setting and government control over major economic sectors (Bahru & Pausewang, 2002).

Dependence on external funding: The overwhelming majority of both international and local Non-Governmental Organisations rely on external sources of funding to run their programme. Government and donors play a key role in promoting Non-Governmental Organisations initiatives which have traditionally weakened the autonomy and effectiveness of Non-Governmental Organisations (Hellinger, 1987a) Non-Governmental Organisations that base their source of funding on governments end up harming the vulnerable, failing to differentiate them and undermining their impendency with the state (Weston, 1994).

Personal interest: Many Non-Governmental Organisations are not domestic, far removed from many social and cultural aspects of society, and many Non-Governmental Organisations tend to retain institutional and personal interests rather than the broader beneficiary (Atsebeha, 2020).

Democratic culture and values: Many Non-Governmental Organisations, especially indigenous, have not internalised democratic cultures. We lack a history of justice and constructive debate and have no media to educate the general public about their acts (g/egziabher, 2002).

Data Quality

The source of performance data is important to the credibility of reported results hence, it is important to incorporate data from a variety of sources to validate findings. Furthermore, while primary data are collected directly by the M&E system for M&E purpose, secondary data are those collected by other organisations for purposes different from M&E (Gebremedhin, Getachew & Amha, 2010). In the design of an M&E system, the objective is to collect indicator data from various sources, including the target population for monitoring project progress (Barton, 1997). Moreover, developing key indicators to monitor outcomes enables managers to assess the degree to which intended or promised outcomes are being achieved (Kusek & Rist, 2004).

2.4 Conceptual Framework

Conceptual frameworks are diagrams that identify and illustrate relationships among relevant organisational, individual and other

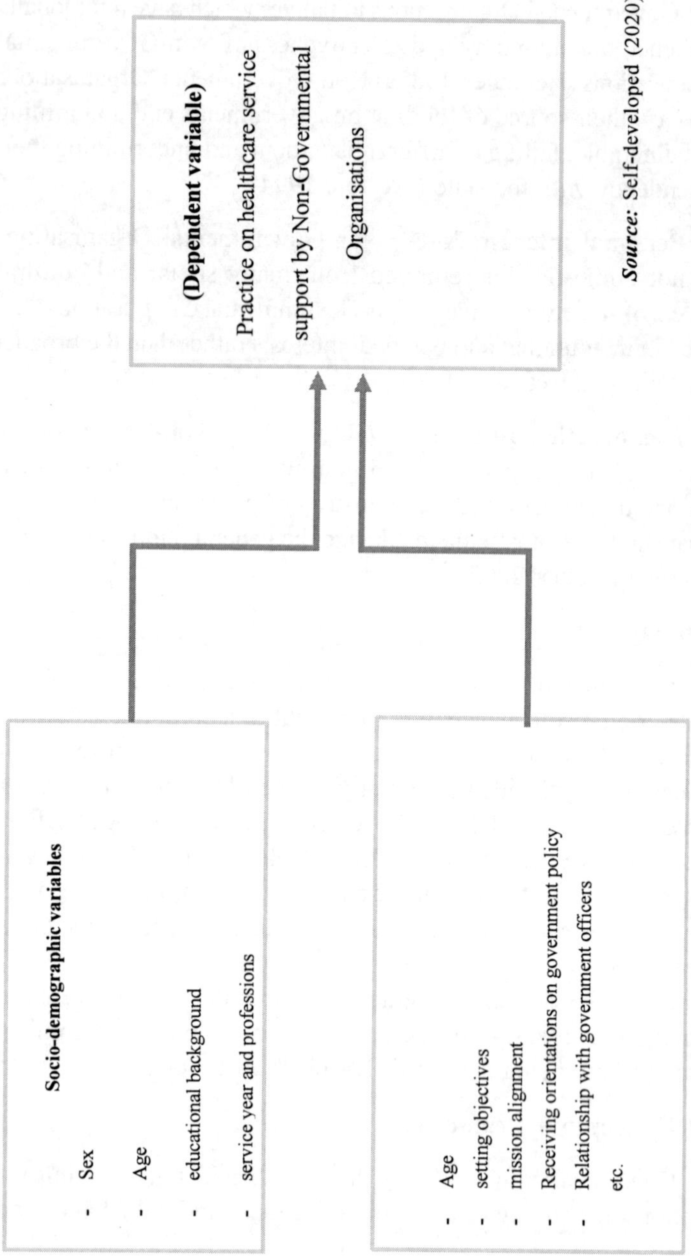

Source: Self-developed (2020)

Fig. 2.1: The Conceptual Framework of Non-Governmental Organisations, Government and Healthcare Service.

factors that may influence a programme and the successful achievement of goals and objectives. They help determine which factors will influence the programme and outline how each of these factors (underlying, cultural, economic socio-political etc.) might relate to and affect the outcomes (Black *et al.*, 2007).

The figure 2.1 shows, the conceptual framework used in this paper shows service providers that include: government and non-governmental organisations and donor agencies. Donor organisations are instrumental sources in health services - training and mobilising capital system building – inputs such as medicines, enhanced quality of life Intervening variables – Political climate – governance – engagement – financing – dynamics of Non-Governmental Organisations – policy – Non-Governmental Organisations dynamics health promotion and prevention of diseases.

3

Research Methodology

3.1 Introduction

According to (Atsebeha, 2020) explained a research methodology refers to a systematic way to solve a problem. It's a method of learning how work is to be carried out. Essentially, the methods by which researchers carry out their task of identifying, explaining and predicting phenomena are called the research methodology. It is also known as the analysis of the methods by which information is acquired. It is supposed to lay down the study work plan.

Therefore, this chapter deals with the methodology that was employed to conduct the study. The study design, target population, sample size and procedures, data collection methods, reliability and validity of data collection instruments, data analysis techniques, and ethical issues were discussed.

3.2 Operational Definition of Variables

The term Non-Governmental Organisation (NGO): can refer to any Non-Governmental Organisation, and different literatures provide different definitions of Non-Governmental Organisations. Worldwide, the list of Non-Governmental Organisations also includes Faith-Based Organisations, religious establishments and political activist groups. The Code of Conduct for Non-Governmental Organisations in Ethiopia articulates a broad distinctiveness of Non-Governmental Organisations as a "voluntary, not for-profit, non-self-serving, non-governmental, non-partisan, and independent organisations or associations" involved in the promotion of social justice and development.

Practice on healthcare service support: this dependent variable was computed from thirteen different practice related questions with Likert scale response.

These questions were transformed to binary variables (4 and 5 becomes good with a value of 1 and 1, 2 and 3 becomes poor with value of 0).

Good practice on healthcare service support: a practice with a value of mean and above from the thirteen computed practice related questions.

Poor practice on healthcare service support: a practice with a value of mean and below from the thirteen computed practice related questions.

Setting an objective: binary variable from Likert scale question (4 and 5 becomes good with a value of 1 and 1, 2 and 3 becomes poor with value of 0).

Having necessary personnel: binary variable from Likert scale question (4 and 5 becomes good with a value of 1 and 1, 2 and 3 becomes poor with value of 0).

Having adequate budget: binary variable from Likert scale question (4 and 5 becomes good with a value of 1 and 1,2 and 3 becomes poor with value of 0).

Conferrable working environment: binary variable from Likert scale question (4 and 5 becomes good with a value of 1 and 1, 2 and 3 becomes poor with value of 0).

Access to government data: binary variable from Likert scale question (4 and 5 becomes good with a value of 1 and 1, 2 and 3 becomes poor with value of 0).

Needs laws and regulations: binary variable from Likert scale question (4 and 5 becomes good with a value of 1 and 1, 2 and 3 becomes poor with value of 0).

Relationship with office: binary variable from Likert scale question (4 and 5 becomes important with a value of 1 and 1, 2 and 3 becomes not important with value of 0).

Receiving orientation on policy: binary variable from Likert scale question (4 and 5 becomes good with a value of 1 and 1, 2 and 3 becomes poor with value of 0).

Licence renewal on time: binary variable from Likert scale question (4 and 5 becomes on time with a value of 1 and 1, 2 and 3 becomes not on time with value of 0).

Alignment of mission: binary variable from Likert scale question (4 and 5 becomes aligned with a value of 1 and 1, 2 and 3 becomes not aligned with value of 0).

3.2.1 Variables

Dependent variable - practice on healthcare service support.

Independent variables-

- **Socio-demographic variables** (sex, age, educational level, position and service year).
- **Opportunities and challenges** (setting an objective, having necessary personnel, having adequate budget, comfortable working environment, access to government data, needs laws and regulations, relationship with office, receiving orientation on policy, licence renewal time and mission alignment).

3.3 Research Approach and Design

3.3.1 Research Approach

This study employed mixed-method research approach which is qualitative and quantitative approaches. According to

(C.R.Kothari, 2004) quantitative research is based on the measurement of quantity or amount and applies to phenomena that can be expressed in terms of quantity, whereas; qualitative research is focused on qualitative phenomena relating to quality or type. So, this study employed a mixed research method of the survey for quantitative and key informant interviews for qualitative research methods. The researcher will collect both quantitative and qualitative data concurrently and then compared the two databases to determine if there is convergence, differences or some combination (Ray, 2019).

3.3.2 Research Design

This study used a cross-sectional survey design that used to make descriptive statistical analyses. The research design allows the researcher to solve the research question in a valid, objective, accurate and economical manner. The study is concerned with describing the characteristics, activities and the situations of individuals, or groups. It requires quantitative, qualitative or mixed approaches (C.R. Kothari, 2004).

3.4 Population and Sample Size

3.4.1 Population

Refers to the entire group of people; event or organisations that a researcher wants to study. The population of this research is the 35 Non-Governmental Organisations operating within Tigray Regional State, Northern Ethiopia. The sample population is all 35 Non-Governmental Organisations that are supporting on the healthcare service, who are implementing or have implemented a healthcare service practice. The population size is therefore finite.

3.4.2 Sample Size

The most important question in the sampling analysis is the size of the sample and how large or small it is. If the sample size is too small, it may not help to achieve the targets, and if it is too big, we may incur huge costs and waste resources. As a general rule, it can be said that the sample must be of the optimal size, i.e.

it should not be too large or too small. Technically, the sample size should be large enough to provide a confidence interval of the desired width and, as such, the sample size should be selected by some logical process before the sample is taken from the universe (Tegegn, 2017). In this cross-sectional survey, the target populations are all 35 Non-Governmental Organisations in Tigray Regional State, Northern Ethiopia. The target population is the total group of people /organisations from which the researcher can obtain information to meet the research objectives.

The sample size was 120 respondents of 35 Non-Governmental Organisations working in supporting the healthcare service in Tigray regional State, Tigray, Northern Ethiopia. The normal point of view is that the size of the sample is the calculated as function of uncertainty, statistical process, strength, and difference. In practice, however, there is a (usually undesirable) tendency to "adjust" other factors, in particular, the difference sought and sometimes the power, in the light of the "practical proprietary requirements for sample size" (Tegegn, 2017).

3.4.3 Sampling Technique

This study was employed with Survey sampling on Non-Governmental Organisations that are working to support the Healthcare service in the study area. The researcher selected these Non-Governmental Organisations, because he finds it helpful to achieve the research objectives. These Non-Governmental Organisations are selected to assess their contribution to the healthcare service delivery, to assess the level of practice, implementation and challenges to verify the common understanding between the government and the Non-Governmental Organisations in the endeavour of healthcare service.

3.5 Data and Instrumentation /Data Collection Techniques

Data collection was made through the use of primary and secondary data collection instruments. The primary data was collected through quantitative and qualitative methods. The data for the quantitative section was collected using a survey questionnaire prepared by addressing all-important variables. A close-ended self-administered questionnaire was prepared in English. Qualitative data was collected using key informants' interviews. The interview was conducted for the government officers working with the Non-Governmental Organisations, Non-Governmental Organisations leaders and workers. Questions for the questionnaire was provided in statement form to show the respondent's attitude from strongly disagree to strongly agree for the Non-Governmental Organisations leaders and workers sought their attitude by putting on a scale from strongly disagree to strongly agree. The interview is prepared in English and translated into Tigrigna for implementation. In line with the interview document reviews was followed the Non-Governmental Organisations offices. The respondents are selected based on their seniority and their familiarity with the issues rose.

3.5.1 Source of Data

The sources of data for this study was only primary sources of data. The primary data was collected through questionnaire for a survey and thorough interview from key informants. To supplement the primary data the researcher will collect information from different sources of secondary data.

3.5.2 Data Collection Instruments

Questionnaires

Questionnaires were the main tool or instrument used to collect data in a descriptive survey research study. Because survey researchers typically study issues and behaviours that change over time, they usually develop new instruments or refine existing ones (Lodico, 2005), so the researcher were distributed a questionnaire to residents in the selected study area. As stated above, the researcher was used structured questionnaires. These questions were included by the researcher as it gives to exhaust the ideas that respondents have about the healthcare service indicators in question.

Key Informant Interview

The interview was used to gather data from the non-government organisations supporting the healthcare service.

3.5.3 Method of Data Analysis and Presentation

The data gathered using the quantitative method was coded and enter to SPSS V 26. It was used to analyse the data to generate the statistics result which was presented as tables, figures and graph. Data collected using qualitative method from key informant interview was analyses thematically by summarising the information gathered from concerned bodies.

3.5.4 Ethical Considerations

Ethical clearance and permission were obtained from the College of Finance Management and Development, Department of Social Security Management, Ethiopian Civil Service University. Before the data collection permissions from the concerned organisations and institutions was asked. During the conducting of interviews, respondents were informed about the purpose and the benefit of the study along with their full right to refuse or completely reject participation. The respondents were informed that their response would be kept confidential and their identity shall not be exposed.

4

Data Presentation, Analysis and Interpretation

4.1 Introduction

Chapter four mainly deals with identifying the major findings and make discussions on these major findings. The study has dealt with various issues in relation to the practice and challenges of Non-Governmental Organisations in supporting the healthcare service in Tigray regional state, Tigray, northern Ethiopia. Some understandings have been created on Non-Governmental Organisations, coordination and support to the healthcare service situation in Tigray. The research has identified the place and position of the Non-Governmental Organisations sector in particular, the contributions of Non-Governmental Organisations in healthcare supports and major challenges that Non-Governmental Organisations face in their operations. Discussions have been made on the findings which emanated from the literature review and the semi-structured interview.

The discussion section mainly focused on major areas such as, the practice and challenges for Non-Governmental Organisations, major practice and challenges of Non-Governmental Organisations and healthcare service situation in Tigray region.

4.2 Response Rate

The study used questionnaires as tools for data collection. The researcher targeted five local Non-Governmental Organisations and 30 International Non-Governmental Organisations, that supports the practice of healthcare service in Tigray Regional States, Northern Ethiopia 2020. For the study, a total of 120 questionnaires were distributed through a hardcopy. Of the total questions 120 were collected through hardcopy which gives 100 percent response rate.

4.3 Demographic Characteristics of the Response (Background Information for the Quantitative Participants)

The study was conducted in 90 (75 percent) males and 30 (25 percent) female respondents. Nearly one-half of the respondents

Table 4.1: Demographic characteristics of the respondents (background information for the quantitative respondents) (N=120)

Characteristics	Categories	Frequency	Percent
Sex of respondent	Male	90	75
	Female	30	25
Educational background of respondent	Diploma	5	4.2
	Degree-BA/BSc	62	51.7
	Master-MA/MSc	53	44.2
Age of respondent	18-25	13	10.8
	26-35	30	25
	36-45	59	49.2
	46-60	17	14.2
	Above 60	1	0.8
Service Year of respondent	1-5	10	8.3
	6-10	33	27.5
	11-20	54	45.0
	Above 20	23	19.2
Position of respondent	Executive	12	10
	Department head	14	11.7
	Supervisor	51	42.5
	Staff	43	35.8

62 (51.7 percent) were first degree holders. Nearly 36 percent were age less than 35 years, and nearly one-half 49.2 percent were 36-45 years of age.

As indicated in Table 4.1, nearly one in three 43 (36 percent) of the respondents had Service year of at most 10 years. With regard to the work position of respondent, 12 (10 percent) were executives, 14 (11.7 percent) department heads, 51 (42.5 percent) Supervisors and the remaining 43 (35.8 percent) were other Staff members (Table 4.1).

Table 4.2: Demographic characteristics of the checklist respondents (background information of the qualitative respondents) (N=29)

Characteristics	Categories	Frequency N=29	Percent
Sex of respondent	Male	26	89.7
	Female	3	10.3
Educational background of respondent	Below Diploma	0	0.0
	Diploma	0	0.0
	Degree-BA/BSc	11	37.9
	Master-MA/MSc	18	62.1
Age of respondent	18-25	2	6.9
	26-35	8	27.6
	36-45	10	34.5
	46-60	9	31.0
Service Year of respondent	1-5	0	0.0
	6-10	6	20.7
	11-20	15	51.7
	Above 20	8	27.6
Position of respondent	Executive	8	27.6
	Department head	7	24.1
	Supervisor	8	27.6
	Staff	6	20.7

As indicated in Table 4.2, 11 (38 percent) of the respondents were first degree holders and the remaining 18 (62 percent) were second degree holders. Among the interviewees, 26 were males and 3 were female respondents.

4.4 Results or Findings

The following findings are inferred from the reviewed literatures and semi-structured interview. The organisations that participated in the interview represent diverse areas of operations, such as relief and rehabilitation, economic and social development, advocacy on human rights issue, women, youth, handicapped and street children. Executive directors, departments heads, programme/project coordinators and in some cases project officers were involved in the interview. In order to protect the anonymity of the names of the persons interviewed they will remain unnamed, but the persons interviewed are coded so as to make the analysis suitable.

4.4.1 Practice of Non-Governmental Organisations on supporting the healthcare service in Tigray, (N=120)

Seventy eight percent (78.8 percent, n=26) of participants in the age group of 26-35 said that Non-Governmental Organisations give good support practice on the healthcare service while, above 55 percent (n=9, 56.3 percent) of the participants in the age group of 46-60 said Non-Governmental Organisations give poor practice on healthcare service support. (P= 0.042). furthermore; above 60 percent (n=69, 62.7 percent) of Non-Governmental Organisations with good level of setting objectives where, in a level of good practice on healthcare service support while 80 percent of Non-Governmental Organisations with poor setting of objectives were in a level of poor practice on healthcare service support (P= 0.015). Almost 70 percent (n=65, 68.4 percent) of the respondents who said good mission alignment had good practice on healthcare service support. On the other hand, above three fourth (76.0 percent, n=19) with poor alignment had poor practice on healthcare service support (P=0.000) (Table 4.3).

Table 4.3: Practice of Non-Governmental Organisations on supporting the healthcare service in Tigray Regional States, Northern Ethiopia, 2020, (N=120)

Variable	Practice on Healthcare Support	
	Poor	Good
	N (%)	N (%)
Sex		
Male	40(44.9)	49 (55.1)
Female	9 (29.0)	22 (77.1)
Educational level		
Diploma	2 (66.7)	1 (33.3)
Degree	22 (34.4)	42 (65.6)
MA/MPH/MS	25 (47.2)	28 (52.8)
Age		
18-25	7 (53.8)	6 (46.2)
26-35	7 (21.2)	26 (78.8)
36-45	26 (44.8)	32 (55.2)
46-60	9 (56.3)	7 (43.8)
Service year		
1-5	3 (30.0)	7 (70.0)
6-10	13 (39.4)	20 (60.6)
11-20	20 (36.4)	35 (63.6)
Above 20	13 (59.1)	9 (40.9)
Position		
Regional coordinator	7 (58.3)	5 (41.7)
Department head	5 (35.7)	9 (64.3)
Supervisor	19 (38.0)	31 (62.0)
Staff	18 (40.9)	26 (59.1)

contd...

Table 4.3: Practice on healthcare service support by Non-Governmental Organisations in Tigray Regional State Northern Ethiopia; 2020 (N=120). (Cont....)

Setting an objective		
Poor	8 (80.0)	2 (20.0)
Good	41 (37.3)	69 (62.7)
Having necessary personnel		
Poor	16 (48.5)	17 (51.5)
Good	33 (37.9)	54 (62.1)
Having adequate budget		
Poor	23 (46.9)	26 (53.1)
Good	26 (36.6)	45 (63.4)
Comfortable working environment		
Poor	17 (50.0)	17 (50.0)
Good	32 (37.2)	54 (62.8)
Access to government data		
Poor	15 (42.9)	20 (57.1)
Good	34 (40.0)	51 (60.0)
Needs laws and regulations		
Not important	14 (46.7)	15 (53.3)
Important	35 (38.90	55 (61.1)
Relationship with office		
Poor	27 (60.0)	18 (40.0)
Good	22 (29.3)	53 (70.7)
Receiving orientation on policy		
Poor	24 (54.5)	20 (45.5)
Good	25 (32.9)	51 (67.1)
License renewal time		
Not on time	21 (48.8)	22 (51.2)
On time	28 (36.4)	49 (63.6)
Alignment of mission		
Not aligned	19 (76.0)	6 (24.0)
Aligned	30 (31.6)	65 (68.4)

Source: SPSS version 26.

4.4.2 Opportunity and Challenges of Non-Governmental Organisations (NGOs)on supporting the healthcare service in Tigray regional state, Northern Ethiopia, 2020, (N=120).

According to the response in the interviews, the study using the qualitative checklist was conducted in 29 respondents. A total of 29 individuals were involved in the interview type of the data, four from Local Non-Governmental Organisations, and 25 were from International Non-Governmental Organisations. Areas of involvement of the Non-Governmental Organisations were Maternal and Reproductive health, health Information, Disease prevention (TB, Malaria, HIV), Nutrition, Water, sanitation and hygiene (WASH). The beneficiaries of the Non-Governmental Organisations were Children, Women, Adolescent and reproductive age group, General population, marginalised and underserved, PLWHIV. With regard to the service duration of the Non-Governmental Organisations, the Non-Governmental Organisations in the study area have served from two years to 16 years (on average seven years). The Non-Governmental Organisations were working in partnership with universities, MOH, Tigray Regional health, Hospitals and Health facilities, other Non-Governmental Organisations, foreign funders, local Non-Governmental Organisations, different sectors (Health, Education, Agriculture, Water), Social and Women's Affairs.

The Major challenges of Non-Governmental Organisations (NGOs) raised from the key informant interview in Tigray regional State were:

1. **Interface problem** – integration /Weak relationship and interface with government.
2. **Poor commitment** – accountability and motivation of staffs and per diem dependence, Dissatisfaction of government health staffs, Low focus by all levels of leaders and excessive meeting.

3. **Resources** - shortages of budgets /Donor depend and less focus / and shortages of lab professionals /Trained staffs turn over due to salary.

4. **System related challenges** - Inappropriate technology, Government structure and weak hand over, Emergency situation and budget shifting, Inadequate data management.

5. **Implementation capacity problem** - at the woreda level, Low capacity government worker at woreda and lower levels.

The freedom Non-Governmental Organisations have in implementing your mission to support the healthcare service

- to technical, financial and logistic support
- to improving the healthcare service
- to contribute in data quality and data use practice betterment
- to improving the awareness and knowledge of health workers
- to capacity and system buildings

With regard to the Non-Governmental Organisations level of flexibility to implement the healthcare service plan, the 21 interviewees stated to be flexible, two somewhat flexible, four highly flexible, and the remaining two stated to be not flexible.

With regard to the acceptance of the Non-Governmental Organisations in the health system, as most projects are designed based on the demand of the Government, there is a high acceptance at all level. The Non-Governmental Organisations Licence renewal and related services are given on time by the health system.

In relation to the governments proclamation 1113/2011 stated about the functions of Non-Governmental Organisations, there was no such a problem encountered by the Non-Governmental Organisations. They respondents stated that they are working accordingly.

As to the level of satisfaction with the service rendered from the government offices working with Non-Governmental Organisations, 21 (70 percent) indicated to be satisfied by the services they get and by the coordination with government and beneficiaries. However, the remaining 8 (30 percent) indicated some issues. The concerns raised were:

- lacks with the issue of sustainability and expectation to pay every time
- Some government staffs are not sensitive to health programmes implementations and they give low focus to Non-Governmental Organisations.
- To improve more professional associations must work hard to hand in order to tackle the challenges in the community.
- Sometimes government organisation are investing their time and every in unnecessary meetings and decision is not working by financial structures and there are ups and downs to facilitate some programmes in collaboration with the government sector heads /staffs.
- The capacity of the government office staff is limited and needs to be strengthened. But the big challenge is staff turnover.

In general, 40.8 (n = 49) of the participants agreed with good practice on healthcare service support by Non-Governmental Organisations (Figure 4.1) below. Furthermore, 91.7 (n = 110) of the participants had agreed with good objective setting before starting their projects. (Table 4.4)

Table 4.4: Opportunity and Challenges of Non-Governmental Organisations (NGOs) on supporting the healthcare service in Tigray Regional States, Northern Ethiopia, 2020 (N = 120)

Variable	Frequency	Percent
Setting an objective		
Poor	10	8.3
Good	110	91.7
Having necessary personnel		
Poor	33	27.5
Good	87	72.5
Having adequate budget		
Poor	49	40.8
Good	71	59.8
Comfortable working environment		
Poor	34	28.3
Good	86	71.7
Access to government data		
Poor	35	29.2
Good	85	79.8
Needs laws and regulations		
Not important	30	25.0
Important	90	75.0
Relationship with office		
Poor	45	37.5
Good	75	62.5
Not on time	43	35.8
On time	77	64.2
Alignment of mission		
Aligned	95	79.8
Not aligned	25	20.8

Source: SPSS version 26.

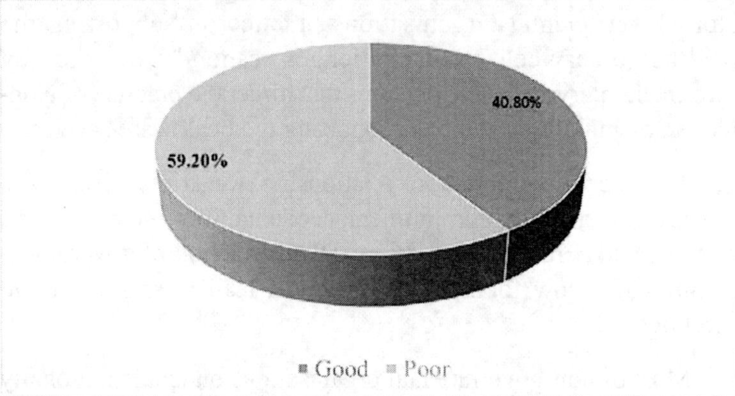

Figure 4.1: The Practice of Non-Governmental Organisations (NGOs) on supporting the healthcare service in Tigray.

Source: SPSS version 26.

4.5 Interpretations and Discussions

4.5.1 The overall practice of Non-Governmental Organisations (NGOs) on supporting the healthcare service

The study found that the practice and challenges of non-governmental organisations on supporting the healthcare service in Tigray. From the information collected from the data collection and findings of challenges above these findings are expressed as follows.

In general, factors affect the practice of Non-governmental organisations on supporting the healthcare service are, age of respondents, setting clear objectives, relationship with the government officials, receiving the orientation on the government policies and mission alignment.

Age of the respondents, with the age 26-35 (78.8 percent), shows that the practice of Non-Governmental Organisations on supporting the healthcare service is good in implementation. In other words, respondents with the age of 46-60, 9 (56.3 percent) shows that the practice of Non-Governmental Organisations on supporting the healthcare service is poor in implementation. Therefore, from this interpretation, workers /leaders with age factor affects the Non-Governmental Organisations practice on supporting the healthcare service. Other challenges respond from the key informant interview questionnaires that affect the practice of Non-Governmental Organisations supporting the healthcare service.

The interface problem, or relationship, weak integration with the government, poor commitment, accountability and motivation of staffs and perdium dependency. Dissatisfaction of government health staffs, low focus by all levels of leaders and executive meetings.

Most of non-governmental organisations budget is regionally depends on the head office. The communication is only by plan and report. They do not have their own and managed budget or the implementation is dependent on the head office, the regional office is only the field office.

There is also, manpower turn over, there is also another challenge to the healthcare service practice supported by the Non-governmental organisations, the shortages of health lab professionals turn over due to low salary.

Challenges with system related challenges like, inappropriate technology, government structure, weak hand over, budget shifting due to emergency situations and, inadequate data management. Implementation capacity problem on the government health workers from the higher to the lower (from bureau to the woreda) level, there is a capacity problem in implementation the healthcare service supported by the non-governmental organisations.

This study is focuses on assessment of the practice and challenges of non-governmental organisations supporting on the healthcare service in Tigray regional States, Northern Ethiopia, 2020. Non-Governmental Organisations are organisations work for not profit, the non-profit organisations in practicing to supports the healthcare service. This report founds the following findings based on the two types of data collection instruments.

Age of Respondents

The age group of 18-26 respondents said that the practice of Non-Governmental Organisations on supporting healthcare service has effectively implemented. On the other hand, the rest of 46-60 age respondents revealed that there is poor practice of implementation in supporting the healthcare service. However, an opposition from the key in formant also revealed that, there is poor relationship among the two organisations, inadequate capacity of workers in supporting healthcare service available in woreda level. Due to such insufficient knowledge of employees, system related challenges are occurred. For example, in appropriate use of technology, government structure, week hand over, emergency situation and budget shifting, and in proper data management are visible.

Setting clear Objective

Findings of the study indicate that there is relatively low capacity of setting objectives, of the total respondents the majority (80 percent) of them expressed there is poor way of preparing working plans (objectives), while the other 20 percent of the sampled also indicated that there is well preparation of setting objectives. In line with above qualitative data, key informants interview also strengthen the idea that there is shortage of budget, shortage of manpower especially, lab professionals as well as more turnover of professional due to less salary and incentives.

According to Health System Development Programme (HSDP, 2004), Non-Governmental Organisations have limited participation in health policy formulation, though there are some indications for a trend for improvement. An informant from one Non-Governmental Organisations said, "Most of us [in Non-Governmental Organisations sector] were not even aware of the health policy and HSDP until years after their ratification." Only few Non-Governmental Organisations participate in the formulation of specific disease control strategies such as that of malaria and HIV/AIDS.

Relationship with offices

The findings from the quantitative data revealed that there is wider gap of communication among government and non-government organisations offices from up to bottom. Of the total samples, 60 percent of them revealed there is poor relationship among the offices, and 40 percent of them also said that there is good relationship among the organisations. On the other direction, the key informants also revealed that there is week communication among the organisations. This show that there is little or no work cooperation and collaboration of tasks related to heath care service support between the offices. Less motivation of staff, dissatisfaction of government staff, weak follow up of leaders towards the work activity rather more time was spent on excessive meetings (CRDA, 2006b).

Though several literatures describe that sectoral policy/ programme participation contributes to democratisation process through participation of citizens, most respondents from Non-Governmental Organisations are not sure of this in the Ethiopian context. The "limited" participation of the target community in the Health Sector Programme in general and the reluctance of Non-Governmental Organisations to advocate on behalf of their target communities are expressed as key reasons for missed opportunity for an added value to be brought by the sector.

Mission Alignment

The findings show that 76 percent of the respondents said there is poor alignment among the two organisations, however, 24 percent of the sample indicated the alignment between them is good. Most interviewee sees this question in many directions as described in the quantitative data, there is poor alignment among the non-government and government organisations, there is high probability to happen numerous problems due to weak alignment, for example, weak relationship, shortage of budget, less task implementation and, system related challenges could be happened

.

Of the 21 key informants asked about the flexibility NGO, 21 of the respondents point out that the NGO are flexible while, two of the respondent indicated to be flexible, four highly flexible, and the last two said not flexible.

The findings also revealed that the level of acceptance of Non-Governmental Organisations in health system, there is high acceptance of Non-Governmental Organisations at all level based on the government demand as well as the licence renewed and related service are given by health system.

According to CRDA, to increase national health spending, the strategic role of Non-Governmental Organisations as partners in achieving universal primary healthcare coverage not only in planning but also implementing healthcare delivery particularly at the woreda level and also emphasises the need to strengthen government-Non-Governmental Organisations collaboration.

The findings from qualitative information also show that most of non-governmental organisations budget is regionally depends on the head office. The communication among them is only by plan and report. They do not have their own and managed budget or the implementation is dependent on the head office, the regional office in only the field office.

As key informant interviews, describe there is also, man power turn over due to various reasons, for example, there is also another challenge to the healthcare service practice supported by the Non-governmental organisations, the shortages of health lab professionals turn over due to low salary (CRDA, 2006b).

Challenges with system related challenges like, inappropriate technology, government structure, weak hand over, budget shifting due to emergency situations and, inadequate data management. Implementation capacity problem on the government health workers from the higher to the lower (from bureau to the woreda) level, there is a capacity problem in implementation the healthcare service supported by the non-governmental organisations.

This study is focuses on assessment of the practice and challenges of non-governmental organisations supporting on the healthcare service in Tigray regional States, Northern Ethiopia, 2020. Non-Governmental Organisations are organisations work for not profit, the non-profit organisations in practicing to supports the healthcare service. This report found the following findings based on the two types of data collection instruments.

Results of the qualitative response of the major challenges faced by the Non-governmental organisations (NGOs) from the key informant interview in Tigray regional State.

Interface problem – integration /weak relationship and interface with government. In other words, however, from other literatures, non-governmental organisations need closed relationship with the government to have a comfortable environment in order to implement their practice on supporting the healthcare service.

Poor commitment, accountability and motivation of staffs and per diem dependence, Dissatisfaction of government health staffs, Low focus by all levels of leaders and Excessive meeting. However, from other literatures, Personal interest: Many Non-Governmental Organisations are not domestic, far removed from many social and cultural aspects of society, and many Non-Governmental Organisations tend to retain institutional and personal interests rather than the broader beneficiary (Atsebeha, 2020).

Resources - shortages of budgets /Donor depend and less focus/ and shortages of lab professionals /Trained staffs turn over due to salary. Shortages of staffs from other study; (Zihindula, Andrew John, Gumede, & Richard Gavin, 2019). However, from other literatures, Weak private sector: in Ethiopia, the private sector is so weak and fragile as to become internal sources of funding for Non-Governmental Organisations, as is the case in many other countries. The private sector is so weak as a result of unfriendly policy setting and government control over major economic sectors (Bahru & Pausewang, 2002). Dependence on external funding: the overwhelming majority of both international and local

Non-Governmental Organisations rely on external sources of funding to run their programme. Government and donors play a key role in promoting Non-Governmental Organisations initiatives which have traditionally weakened the autonomy and effectiveness of Non-Governmental Organisations (Hellinger, 1987a) Non-Governmental Organisations that base their source of funding on governments end up harming the vulnerable, failing to differentiate them and undermining their impendency with the state (Weston, 1994).

System related challenges: Inappropriate technology, Government structure and weak hand over, Emergency situation and budget shifting, Inadequate data management. However, from other literatures many Non-Governmental Organisations, especially indigenous, have not internalised democratic cultures. We lack a history of justice and constructive debate and have no media to educate the general public about their acts (g/egziabwher, 2002).

Implementation capacity problem - at the woreda level, Low capacity government worker at woreda and lower levels. However, from other literatures, there is Capacity limitation significant limitation of the capacity of indigenous Non-Governmental Organisations. Limiting human resources and budget constraints are key features of local Non-Governmental Organisations. The lack of access to resources, physical assets, and human capital is characteristic of Ethiopian Non-Governmental Organisations.

5

Conclusion and Recommendation

5.1 Introduction

This study aimed to investigate the practice and challenges of Non-Governmental Organisations programme in supporting the healthcare service in Tigray Region, by employing mixed methods design and collecting data using interviews and, questionnaires. It came up with a number of insights presented, interpreted and discussed in Chapter four. This last chapter summarises the major findings that emerged from the analysis of the qualitative and quantitative data collected for the study. Finally, based on the findings, it draws conclusions and recommendations.

5.2 Conclusion

The practice and challenges of Non-Governmental Organisations (NGOs) in supporting the healthcare service in the study was low. Where, respondents age, setting an objective, relationship with government officials, receiving orientation about the government policy and mission alignment are different factors. Furthermore, the interface problem, poor commitment of the government workers, resources like budgets and professionals and trained staffs, system related challenges (government structure, inadequate data access, weak hand over, budget shifting due to emergency situation) and implementation capacity problem were reflected challenges from the participants.

Therefore, the government should create a favorable environment for the non-governmental organisations so as to give the contribution in supporting the healthcare service practice.

Non-Governmental Organisations practice in the areas of healthcare service, is extraordinary but based on the government's orientation and interface in working with governments plan, it is less. The previous trend of Non-Governmental Organisations on supporting the healthcare service focusing on sustainable relief. They began collaborating with the government development plan. Due to lack of resource and collaboration with government, Non-Governmental Organisations could not clearly report their performance and understand their local context. Most Non-Governmental Organisations get their operational budget from foreign source due to this they depend on their donor's plan. Generally speaking, the collaboration and net-working activity is not satisfactorily implemented. There are misunderstandings on the legal and policy issues between the Non-Governmental Organisations and the government. As it is presented in the analysis, the classification of activities between administrative and operational are not clearly stated. Even if proclamation 1113/2011 is not clear to the Non-Governmental Organisations those are supporting the healthcare service in Tigray. The reason that they raise is because of the office of field cite office, their communication is by plan and report. Most of the Non-Governmental Organisations did not know about the proclamation and the amount of budget they facilitate. The agency faced problem in human resource and technical capacity.

Finally, the practice of non-governmental organisations on supporting the healthcare service is poor by N = 71 (59.20 percent) and good by N = 49 (40.80 percent). So, the government should create a comfortable environment to the non-governmental organisations to support the healthcare service effectively and also, the non-governmental organisations should assess and solve the threats those are raised as challenges to the healthcare service practice supported by them.

5.3 Recommendations

Recommendations are offered for Non-Governmental Organisations, governments, donors, and future research including studying the organisational effectiveness and sustainability of these partnerships to deliver effective and efficient health outcomes to recommend universal best practices in healthcare service.

As it is presented in the above results, most Non-Governmental Organisations are getting their fund from few sources of which the majority are foreign sources. Non-Governmental Organisations should plan on the sustainability of their projects by soliciting funds from different sources. Strengthening local resource mobilisation is crucial. In line with that, by building the local capacity they have to work on avoiding dependency mentality. Non-Governmental Organisations should involve in income generation activities. They have also need to expand their donor base. To have income generation scheme helps to minimise total dependence on foreign funds. Non-Governmental Organisations should conduct base line survey and evaluation to clearly understand the local context, to improve their service and to clearly report their performance. Working closely and in collaboration with different partners and stakeholders is extremely essential to minimalise duplication of efforts and ensure service quality and sustainability. Non-Governmental Organisations should strengthen the good effort started with regard to collaboration. To create a common understanding on legal and policy issues discussion panels are needed between the government and the Non-Governmental Organisations. The government once in a while gives orientation on legal and policy issues and this should continue to avoid confusion and misunderstanding and to get an input from all stakeholders even to improve some legal and policy issues. Non-Governmental Organisations should comply with the laws and policies of the country. The government should strengthen the capacity of the established agency, so that to render best service as much as possible.

5.4 Recommendation for Non-Governmental Organisations (NGOs)

It is an opportunity provides potential for Non-Governmental Organisations to raise funds from external funder and other donors.

- Identify and analysing the existing problem or well doing of the gap.
- The Non-Governmental Organisations should focus on high demand or profitable business.
- Identify and share best practice on the healthcare service improvement.
- Create strong Stake Holderness and generating their income as the private models like Shareholder Company.
- Capacitate their internal/the staff.
- Collaborate with in different Non-Governmental Organisations to form partners to facilitate their practice on the healthcare service.
- Non-Governmental Organisations should be focusing of their internal resource for long-term financial suitability.
- Non-Governmental Organisations will amended their strategic plan.

5.5 Suggestions for Further Research

Due to the distinct lack of related researches about the assessment of practice and challenges of Non-Governmental Organisations in supporting the healthcare service, it seems premature at this stage to make any suggestion particularly on policy issues. Instead of more value would be additional research on the subject area. The following areas are suggested for further research:

Assessment of practice and challenges of Non-Governmental Organisations on supporting the healthcare service in Tigray Regional State, 2020.

(i) Further research to identify the governmental side. That is how the Non-governmental organisations are implementing the support to the healthcare service.

(ii) Further research would be required to determine the actual impact of in practicing the healthcare service support by local and international Non-Governmental Organisations executed projects in the region.

References

Anurag Priyadarshee. (2010). *Microfinance, Social Protection and Poverty: Challenges and Opportunities for Service Delivery in India Table of Contents.*

Atsebeha, K. G. (2020). *Assessment on practice and challenges of non-governmental organisations in providing healthcare service in Ethiopia.*

Bahru, Z., & Pausewang, S. (2002). *Ethiopia: the challenge of democracy from below*. Nordiska Afrikainstitutet; Forum for Social Studies, Addis Ababa.

Black, M. M., Dubowitz, H., Krishnakumar, A., Starr, R. H., Vohr, Poindexter, B. B., … Society, S. (2007). Persistent beneficial effects of breast milk ingested in the neonatal intensive care unit on outcomes of extremely low birth weight infants at 30 months of age. *Pediatrics*. https://doi.org/10.1111/j.1469-7610.2007.01752.x

C.R. Kothari. (2004). *Research Methodology* (second rev).

Campbell. (1996). *University of Graduate Institute of International Development and Applied Economics By Ayele Angelo Ago Dissertation Prepared in partial fulfilment of the requirements for MA Degree in Social Development and Sustainable Livelihoods, University of Reading.*

Charity & Society Agency. (2017). The role of NGOs in corporate environmental responsibility practice: evidence from Ethiopia.

International Journal of Corporate Social Responsibility, *2*(1). https://doi.org/10.1186/s40991-017-0013-0

Cheston S., & Kuhn, L. (2002). *Empowering Women Through Microfinance.*

Christian Relief & Development Association. (2014). *The Contribution of Non-Governmental Organisations in Delivery of Basic Health Services in Partnership with Local Government: A.* https://doi.org/10.13140/RG.2.1.3772.6886

Clark. (2004). Assessment of Income Generation Practices and Challenges among NGOs operating in Addis Ababa: The case of Kolfe Keranyo and Lideta Sub-cities.

CRDA. (2006a). *Assessment of the operating invironment for civil society in Ethiopia.*

CRDA. (2006b). *The participation of NGOs/CSOs in the Health Sector Development Programme of Ethiopia.*

Desalegn. (2008). *Ethiopia Service Provision Assesement plus Survey 2014.*

g/egziabher. (2002). *The role of civil society in democratisation.*

GTZ. (2011). *National Social Protection Strategy*. (January).

Hellinger. (1987a). *NGOs and Donors*. (December).

Hellinger. (1987b). *NGOs and the large aid donor.*

Henwood, Nicholson, R. & S. (2005). *Qualitative Research Practice.14*(2), 47. https://doi.org/10.18352/jsi.39

https//:www.chsa.gov.et. (2009). Strengthening health systems: Strengthening health systems: In *Health (San Francisco).*

Kassa, K. & S. (2015). The Situation of Street Children in Urban Centers of Ethiopia and the Role of NGOs in Addressing their Socio-Economic Problems: The Case of Hawassa City. *International Journal of Academic Research in Education and Review*, *3*(3), 45–57. https://doi.org/10.14662/IJARER2015.012

Lewis, Davis & Kanji, N. (2009). *The widespread challenges of NGOs in developing countries: Case studies from Iran*. *6*(September), 197–202. https://doi.org/10.5897/NGOJ11.014

Lodico. (2005). *College of Business and Economics School of Commerce Assessment of Neighborhood Indicators in Addis Ababa Condominium Housing Projects to Enhance Sustainable Urban College of Business and Economics School of Commerce, Department of Project Management Assess*.

Mathew Brown. (2009). Non-governmental organisations and development. In *Non-Governmental Organisations and Development*. https://doi.org/10.4324/9780203877074

Norad. (2005). *The study of the impact of FORUT*.

Pluto. (1996). Non-governmental organisations and development. In *Non-Governmental Organisations and Development*. https://doi.org/10.4324/9780203877074

Rajeev, D. (2016). *Role of Non-Governmental Organisations in Healthcare Sector of India*. https://doi.org/10.13140/rg.2.2.30420.19845

Ray, R. (2019). Designing and Conducting Mixed Methods Research [Book Review]. *Qualitative Research Journal*, *7*(2), 90–91. https://doi.org/10.3316/qrj0702090

Richard, G. & Wamai. (2004). *Recent International Trends in NGO Health System Organisation, Development and Collaborations with Government in Transforming Healthcare Systems*.

Richard, G. & Wamai. (2009). *Reviewing Ethiopian health system development*.

Sunshant. (2010). *The perception of stake holders on the role of NGOs in development.*

Tegegn, G. (2017). *Assessment of Income Generation Practices and Challenges among NGOs operating in Addis Ababa: The case of Kolfe Keranyo and Lideta Sub-cities.*

Turner & Hulme. (2008). *University of Graduate Institute of International Development and Applied Economics By Ayele Angelo Ago Dissertation Prepared in partial fulfilment of the requirements for MA Degree in Social Development and Sustainable Livelihoods, University of Reading.*

UNICEF. (2017a). *Lessons from Ghana: A Role for Social Protection Investments to Support Food and Nutrition Security.* (February). Retrieved from www.csis.org

UNICEF. (2017b). *Maternity protection and workers with family responsibilities in the formal and informal economy of Ghana. Practices , gaps and measures for improvement.*

USAID. (2009). Successes in social protection: What lessons can be learned? *Canadian Journal of Development Studies.* https://doi.org/10.1080/02255189.2011.647446

USAID. (2017). *UNICEF Annual Report 2017 Ethiopia.* Retrieved from https://www.unicef.org/about/annualreport/files/Bangladesh_2017_COAR.pdf

Weston. (1994). *Reflection on NGO sustainable livelihood.*

World Bank. (2000). *World development report.*

Zewdie & Pausewan. (2002). *The challenges of democracy in Ethiopia.*

Zihindula, G., Andrew John, R., Gumede, D. M., & Richard Gavin, M. (2019). A review on the contributions of NGOs in addressing the shortage of healthcare professionals in rural South Africa. *Cogent Social Sciences*, Vol. 5. https://doi.org/10.1080/23311886.2019.1674100

Index